HAYFA BERGAOUI
Yessine Belhadj Taher
Imen Ghadhab

SCREENING FOR GENITAL STREPTOCOCCUS B CARRIAGE IN THE THIRD TRIMESTER

HAYFA BERGAOUI
Yessine Belhadj Taher
Imen Ghadhab

SCREENING FOR GENITAL STREPTOCOCCUS B CARRIAGE IN THE THIRD TRIMESTER

ScienciaScripts

Contents

INTRODUCTION

Group B Streptococcus (GBS), or Streptococcus Agalactiae, has been identified as the main cause of severe bacterial infections in mothers, fetuses and neonates (1). This bacterium intermittently colonises the vaginal cavity of many women, who are considered "healthy" carriers (2). Transmission occurs via the ascending route or when passing through the vaginal tract, and very rarely via hematogenesis (3).

GBS colonises pregnant women in all regions of the world, with the prevalence of carriage varying from one region to another, with a global estimate, according to a 2017 study by Neal J Russel et al, of between 11% and 35% and a mean (M) of 18% (4). It may be chronic or intermittent, and is more prevalent in the last trimester (5). Its transmission is maximal at the time of delivery (1).

A study carried out in Morocco in the Marrakech region published in 2016 found that the prevalence of GBS carriage in pregnant women was 20.2% (6).

The last study carried out in our department in Tunisia in 2010 found a GBS carriage prevalence of 7.3% in the Monastir region (7).

In view of the extent of maternal colonisation, the pathogenicity of this bacterium and the complications that may arise, and in order to reduce maternal-foetal transmission of GBS, recommendations have been put forward. These include those based solely on risk factors and those based on systematic screening of all pregnant women, ideally between 35 and 37 weeks' amenorrhoea (SA), followed by prophylactic intrapartum antibiotic treatment for colonised women. The aim of these recommendations is to reduce colonisation of newborns by at least 80%(3).

Another preventive strategy against early-onset invasive GBS disease is vaccination of pregnant women, which could improve the trans-placental transfer of anti-GBS antibodies to Icetus (8).

Very few Tunisian studies have focused on this subject, so we set out to evaluate the proportion of streptococcus B in daily practice in our maternity hospital through a cross-sectional study with the following objectives:

- To determine the prevalence of vaginal carriage of streptococcus B in the third trimester of pregnancy.

- Identify the main risk factors involved in portage.
- Defining a screening strategy for streptococcus B.
- To determine the diagnostic and therapeutic means of vaginal carriage of GBS.

PATIENTS AND METHOD

This is a descriptive and analytical cross-sectional study conducted at the Monastir Maternity and Neonatology Centre over a 5-month period from October 2018 to February 2019.

1. Study population

The study involved a sample of 330 women with a vaginal swab (VS) for group B streptococcus from 34SA.

The inclusion criteria were: All asymptomatic parturients with a vaginal swab from 34SA who gave birth in our maternity hospital. In order to optimise selection bias, we recruited our patients at the outpatient clinic during their antenatal consultations.

The non-inclusion criteria were: All parturients:

- Not having a vaginal swab
- Not having given birth in our maternity hospital
- Presenting a clinical point of call :

■ leucorrhea

■ uterine contractions (threat of premature labour or woman in labour)

■ pyelonephritis gravidarum (PNA g) or premature rupture of membranes (RPM).

- Having received antibiotic treatment 15 days previously.

II. Protocol

We tested for streptococcus B by taking a vaginal swab at the antenatal clinic between 34 and 38 weeks' gestation.

In accordance with the recommendations of the Agence Nationale d'Accreditation et d'Evaluation en Sante (ANAES) published in September 2001, the vaginal swab was taken in the examination room, with the parturient in the gynaecological position, using a swab without the use of a speculum, sweeping the lower third of the vagina as far as the vestibule and the vulva, without reaching the posterior vaginal pouch and without taking an associated rectal swab.

The sample was delivered rapidly to the bacteriology laboratory, without any preservation medium, within half an hour.

Labour and delivery were managed in the usual way, with antibiotics prescribed during labour in patients with risk factors:

- Premature rupture of membranes lasting more than 12 hours.
- Maternal fever during labour above 38.5°C.

These women were systematically given "amoxicillin-clavulanic acid" at a dose of : 1g every 8 hours until delivery after an infectious work-up.

Patients labelled as streptococcus B positive were given intravenous antibiotic therapy from the start of labour, based on :

Ampicillin: 2g initial loading dose then 1g every 4 hours

Erythromycin: 500 mg every 6 hours if allergic to penicillin.

This antibiotic prophylaxis protocol could be modified according to :

- Antibiotic susceptibility test results
- Availability of the chosen molecule

Newborns of mothers with GBS who had undergone vaginal delivery were to benefit from peripheral sampling.

III. Parameters studied

We have considered the following parameters:

- Socio-demographic characteristics. (age, origin, gender, parity...)
- Gyneco-obstetrical antecedents. (MFIU, FCS, DG, MAP)
- Medical history. (diabetes...)
- The course of the current pregnancy and complications. (gestational diabetes, hypertension, PNAg, IUGR, etc.)
- How the work is carried out. (fever, RPM...)
- Characteristics of the newborn. (birth weight, Apgar, etc.)

IV. Ethics

Our study does not pose any ethical problems as it does not affect either ethical principles or the personal lives of patients. Authorisation from the head of department at the Monastir Maternity and Neonatology Centre is required to access the data.

V. Data sources

The data for our study were collected using the Data Collection Form (**see appendix**), which came from :

- Obstetrical records
- Operating reports.
- Liaison or transfer forms.
- Hospital records.

VI. Statistical analysis

Data were entered using Statistical Package for the Social Science Software (SPSS) version 23.0.

With regard to descriptive statistics, quantitative variables were represented by means (M) and standard deviations (SD) for variables following the normal distribution or by medians (Me) and interquartile range (IIQ) for non-Gaussian variables. Qualitative variables were represented by the numbers and frequencies. The normality of quantitative variables was verified by the Shapiro-Wilk test if the sample size was < 50 and by the Kolmogorov-Smirnov test if the sample size was larger.

For the univariate analysis of independent samples in search of associated factors, we performed the Chi-square test for qualitative variables. For quantitative variables, we performed the Mann-Whitney U test for non-Gaussian quantitative variables and the Student t test for variables following the normal distribution.

A significance level of less than 5% was used for all statistical tests, with a confidence interval (CI) set at 95%.

We then performed a multivariate analysis using binary logistic regression (method entree) to determine the risk factors for streptococcal carriage in pregnant women. Independent variables were included in the regression model when their significance level was less than 0.2.

RESULTS

I. Descriptive study of the population studied

1. Socio-demographic characteristics

The average age of the population studied was 31 ± 5.5 years, with extremes ranging from 17 to 47 years. The level of education was higher in more than a third of cases. More than half of the women were of urban origin.

Table I: Socio-demographic characteristics of the population studied

	Workforce (n=330)	Percentage (%)
Age (years)		31 ± 5,52
School level		
Illiterate	6	1,8
Primary	90	27,3
Secondary	113	34,2
Superior	121	36,7
Habitat		
Rural	141	42,7
Urban	189	57,3
Profession		
Housewives	150	45,5
Worker	114	34,5
Other	66	20
Weight (Kg)		82 [71,5 - 91,5]

2. Background

2.1. Medical history

A history of diabetes was noted in 27 patients (8.2%). Dysthyroidism was noted in 2 patients. Chronic hypertension was noted in 6 patients.

2.2. Gyneco-obstetrical history

The gestational age ranged from 1 to 9 with a median of 2 [1-3].

Parity ranged from 1 to 6 with a median of 2 [1-3]. Primiparity was noted in 35.5% of cases.

With regard to gynaecological-obstetric antecedents, we noted that 73 patients, i.e. 22.1% of cases, had undergone miscarriage.

2.3. *water II: Medical and gynaecological-obstetric antecedents of the population studied*

	Number (n=330)	Percentage (%)
Diabetes	27	8,2
Dysthyroidism	2	0,6
Chronic hypertension	6	1,8
Spontaneous miscarriages	73	22,1
Extrauterine pregnancy (EP)	7	2,1
Death per partum	1	0,3
Voluntary termination of pregnancy (IVG)	20	6,1
Therapeutic termination of pregnancy (ITG)	3	0,9
MAP	1	0,3
Mort 1%'tale in utero (MFIU)	9	2,7
Neonatal death	4	1,2
Streptococcus carriage	2	0,6
Gestite		2 [1-3]
Primigeste	91	27,6
Multigeste	239	72,4
Parite		2 [1-3]
Primipare	117	35,5
Multipare	213	64,5

3. Pregnancy in progress

Sixteen patients (4.8%) had a multiple pregnancy, including two triplets (0.6%). Complications arising during pregnancy:

• Gestational diabetes (GD) was noted in 92 patients (27.9%). Approximately one third (29.3%) of diabetic patients were on insulin.

• Pre-term and post-PV PMR were noted in 17 patients (5.2%), who had undergone PV before PMR.

• Intrauterine growth retardation (IUGR) was noted in 51 patients (15.6%).

• PAD and gestational ANP were noted in 3.3% (11 patients) and 3.6% (12 patients) of cases respectively, and these patients had undergone PV before the onset of these two complications.

• Gestational arterial hypertension (g-arterial hypertension) was noted in 20 patients (6.1%).

• MFIU was noted in 8 patients (2.4%).

Table III: Complications occurring during pregnancy

	Workforce (n=330)	Percentage (%)
Gestational diabetes	92	27,9
RPM before and after completion of the PV	17	5,2
IUGR	51	15,6
MAP after completion of the PV	11	3,3
NAP after completion of the PV	12	3,6
Pregnancy-induced hypertension	20	6,1
MFIU	8	2,4

4. Term of delivery

The median term of delivery was 38 [34.4 - 39.5] and prematurity was noted in 23.3% of cases.

5. Work in progress

5.1. Working hours

The median working time was 3 hours [0 hours -6 hours], with extremes ranging from 0 to 48 hours.

5.2. Duration of the opening of the reuf

The average opening time was 2 hours [Hour - 11 hours]. The mean was 15.2 hours, with extremes ranging from 0 to 360 hours. RPM (>12 hours) was noted in 72 patients (21.8%).

5.3. Fever

A fever was noted in 14 patients, i.e. in 4.2% of cases.

6. The birth process

6.1. Delivery route

The majority of women (60% of cases) had given birth vaginally.

85 women (25.8% of cases) had given birth by scheduled caesarean section and 47 women had given birth by emergency caesarean section.

Table IV: Routes of delivery in the population studied

	Number (n=330)	Percentage (%)
VB	198	60
Cesarean section scheduled	85	25,8
Emergency Caesarean section	47	14,2

6.2. APGAR score

The APGAR score had a median of 10 [9-10]. MFIU was noted in 2.4% of cases.

6.3. Birth weight

The median birth weight was 3230g [2800g-3700g].

6.4. Presentation

The presentations of childbirth observed in the population studied were distributed as follows:

- Cephalic presentation: 318 cases (96.4%).
- Seat presentation: 10 cases (3%).
- Transverse presentation: 2 cases (0.6%).

II. Prevalence and carriage of streptococcus in pregnant women

1. Prevalence of streptococcus carriage in pregnant women

In our study population, 86 pregnant women (26.1%) had a positive PV.

The prevalence of streptococcus B in pregnant women in our study was 8.8% (29 patients).

Table V: Vaginal sampling characteristics of the population studied

	Number (n=330)	Percentage (%)
Positive PV		
No	244	73,9
Yes	86	26,1
Streptococcus B carriage		
No	301	91,2
Yes	29	8,8

2. Bacteriological study of streptococcal carriage in pregnant women

2.1. Antibiotic prophylaxis

Of the 29 women with a positive antibiogram, 22 were put on antibiotic prophylaxis (75.8%). Of the seven patients who had not received prophylactic antibiotic treatment, five had given birth by cesarean section and two had given birth vaginally but had no PV results available.

2.2. Molecules used in antibiotic therapy

The molecule of choice for antibiotic prophylaxis was Totapen in 77.22% of cases. Five women had an allergy to penicillin and were treated with erythromycin.

Table VI: Molecules used in the study population

Family	Molecules	Workforce	Percentage
Penicillin	Totapen	17	77,22
Macrolides	Erythromycin	5	22,73

III. Bi-variee analytical study

1. Streptococcal B carriage and socio-demographic characteristics

Our bi-variate study involved two groups, the first comprising 301 parturients with a negative or positive PV for a germ other than GBS, and the second group containing 29 women with a positive PV for streptococcus B.

With regard to socio-demographic characteristics, patients of rural origin were more likely to be carriers of streptococcus B than patients of urban origin, with a statistically significant difference (p=0.027).

Table VII: Comparison of socio-demographic characteristics as a function of streptococcus B carriage

	Group1 Streptococcus B - (n=301)	Group 2 Streptococcus B+ (n :29)	P
Age (years)	31 [27-34]	30 [28-37]	0,301
School level			
Illiterate	6	0	0,726
Primary	80	10	
Secondary	104	9	
Superior	111	10	
Habitat			
Rural	123	18	**0,027**
Urban	178	11	
Profession			
Housewives	136	14	0,749
Woman in work	165	15	
Weight	83[71,5-92]	78,5[71-89,5]	0,572

2. Streptococcus B carriage and medical and obstetric-gynaecological antecedents

With regard to medical and gynaecological-obstetric antecedents, we noted that the antecedent of diabetes and the antecedent of streptococcus B carriage exposed women to a higher risk of being a streptococcus B carrier, with a statistically significant difference ($p<10^{-3}$ and p=0.007 respectively).

Table VIII: Comparison of medical and obstetric-gynecological antecedents between the two groups

	Groupe1 Streptococcus -	Group 2 Streptococcus +	P
Diabetes	12	15	$<10^{-3}$ ***
Spontaneous miscarriages	67	6	0,846
EUS	7	0	0,522
Death per partum	1	0	0,912
ABORTION	18	2	0,542
ITG	3	0	0,758
MAP	1	0	0,912
MFIU	9	0	0,432
Neonatal death	4	0	0,691
History of streptococcal B carriage	from 0	2	**0,007*****
Gestite	2[1 - 3]	2[2 - 4]	
primigeste	87	4	0,297
multigeste	214	25	0,082
Parite	2[1-3]	2[2-3]	
primiparous	111	6	0,072*
multipare	190	23	0,082*

3. Streptococcus B carriage and the course of the current pregnancy

With regard to the characteristics of the pregnancy in progress, only the complication of IUGR was associated with the carriage of streptococcus B, with a statistically significant difference (p=0.046).

Table IX: Comparison of the characteristics of the current pregnancy

	Groupe1 Streptococcus -	Group 2 Streptococcus +	P
Twin pregnancies	14	0	0,268

Triplet pregnancy	2	0	0,832
Gestational diabetes	87	5	0,181
IUGR	50	1	**0,046****
RPM before term and after PV production	16	1	0,548
MAP after completion of the PV	10	1	0,642
PNAgravidique after PV production	11	1	0,715
HTA	19	1	0,458

4. Streptococcus B carriage and term of delivery

The term distribution was identical in both groups. No statistically significant correlation was found between prematurity and streptococcus B carriage.

Table X: Streptococcus B carriage and term of delivery

	Groupe1 Streptococcus B -	Group 2 Streptococcus B +	P
Prematurity (< 36SA)	77	0	0,577
Term of delivery	38,4 [36,4 - 39,4]	39,6 [39,2- 40]	0,188

5. Carrying streptococcus B and the labour process

5.1. Working hours

The median duration of labour in the group of pregnant women with streptococcus B was 5.5 hours [4 hours-7 hours]. The distribution of the duration of labour was identical between the two groups (p=0.139).

5.2. Duration of the opening of the reuf

The median time to open the egg in the group of pregnant women carrying streptococcus B was 1.5 hours [0-7 hours]. There was no significant difference in the time taken to open the uterus between the two groups (p=0.534). RPM was not related to streptococcus B carriage (p=0.611).

Table XI: Streptococcus B carriage and duration of labour and opening of the uterus

	Groupe1	Group 2	p

	Streptococcus B -	Streptococcus B +	
Working hours	1,5 [0-5]	5,5 [4-7]	0,139
Duration of opening I'CL'llf	2 [0-11]	1,5 [0-7]	0,534

5.3. Fever

Fever was noted in 14 patients. These patients belonged to the Streptococcus B group (p=0.917).

6. Carrying streptococcus B and the delivery process

With regard to the characteristics of the delivery, no factor was associated with streptococcus B carriage.

Table XII: Comparison of delivery characteristics

	Groupe1 Streptococcus -	2P Group Streptococcus +	
Delivery route			
VB	177	21	0,153*
Cesarean section programmed	80	5	0,272
Emergency Caesarean section	44	3	0,383
Neonatal weight	3200[2800 3700]	3475[3025 3575]	0,449
APGAR	10[9-10]	10[9-10]	0,823
MFIU	8	0	0,475

7. Carrying streptococcus B and hospitalisation of newborns

Of the four newborn babies hospitalised from a mother carrying streptococcus B, three presented with acute foetal distress (AFS) and the fourth had a maternal-foetal infection (MFI).

There was no association between the carriage of streptococcus B and hospitalisation of the newborn.

Table XIII: Carriage of streptococcus B and hospitalisation of newborns

Hospitalization	Groupe1 Streptococcus B -	Group 2 Streptococcus B	P
Yes	64	4	0,342
No	237	25	

IV. Multivariate analysis: Risk factors for streptococcal B carriage

Logistic regression based on the initial bi-variate analysis identified that living in a rural environment exposed pregnant women to a 2.7 risk of streptococcal B carriage (p=0.033) and that a history of diabetes exposed pregnant women to a 27.6 risk of streptococcal B carriage (p<10).[-3]

Table XIV: Risk factors for streptococcus B carriage

	P	OR	Confidence interval
Housing in rural areas	0,033	2,709	[1,084-6,764]
History of diabetes	■10 3	27,595	[10,498-72,536]

V. Main results

A total of 330 patients were included in the study. The mean age was 30.9 ± 5.5 years, with extremes ranging from 17 to 47 years. More than half of the women were of urban origin. A history of diabetes was noted in 8.2% of cases. Gestational age and parity had a median of 2 [1-3]. Primiparity was noted in 35.5% of cases. FCS was predominant in 73 patients, i.e. 22.1% of cases. Sixteen patients had multiple pregnancies, two of which were triplets. Gestational diabetes was noted in 27.9% of cases. 29.3% of diabetic patients were on insulin. 5.2% of women had preterm PMR after PV. There were 51 IUGRs (15.6% of cases). Prematurity was noted in 24% of cases. 8 cases of MFIU were noted, i.e. 2.4% of cases.

The prevalence of streptococcus B carriage among pregnant women in our study was 8.8%. Of the 29 women with a positive antibiogram for streptococcus B, 22 were put on prophylactic antibiotic therapy.

The molecule of choice for antibiotic prophylaxis was Totapen in 77.22% of cases. Five women with penicillin allergy were treated with erythromycin.

Four newborn babies born to mothers carrying streptococcus B were admitted to hospital.

The factors associated with streptococcus B carriage were :

- Rural origin (p=0.027).
- History of diabetes (p<10 $)^{-3}$
- Previous streptococcus B carriage (p=0.007).
- IUGR (p=0.046).

The risk factors for streptococcus B carriage after logistic regression were :

- living in rural areas OR = 2.7; CI [1.084 -6.764], p=0.033
- history of diabetes OR = 27.6; CI [10.498-72.536], p<10 $.^{-3}$

DISCUSSION

I. Prevalence

GBS colonises pregnant women in all regions of the world, with the prevalence of carriage varying from region to region, with a global estimate of between 11% and 35%, and an average of 18% (4).

In our study, asymptomatic carriage of group B streptococcus in full-term parturients was **8.8%**.

Table XV: Frequency of GBS carriage in the literature according to sampling site

Authors	Years	Collection site	prevalence	country
Skhiri I (7)	2010	V	7.3%	Tunisia
Shirazi M (9)	2014	V	4.9%	Iran
KT Mitima (10)	2014	V	20%	DR Congo
M Kunze(11)	2015	V or V+R	18.5%	Germany
Arain F R (12)	2015	V+R	24%	Arabia Saudi Arabia
L Matsiane Lekalan(13)	2015	V+R	48.2%	South Africa
K. Le Doare(14)	2016	V+R	33.7%	Gambia
Bassir A(6)	2016	V	20.2%	Morocco
MoraledaC (15)	2017	V+R	24%	Morocco
Mahrane S (16)	2017	V+R	22.6%	Algeria

V: Vaginal R: Rectal

A meta-analysis published by Oxford University in England in 2017 by Neal J. Russell et al (4) detailed the prevalence of GBS carriage in different continents and regions worldwide. An adjusted estimate of maternal GBS colonisation worldwide was 18%. Prevalence was highest in the Caribbean at 34% and lowest in Melanesia at 2%; Europe, North America and Australia had a similar prevalence of 15% to 21%, with a prevalence in Southern Africa of 25% and apparently lowest in West Africa 14%; Central America 10%; South, South-East and East Asia 9% to 12%.

In Germany, the number of pregnant women who were asymptomatic carriers of GBS was estimated at 18.5% in a study carried out in 2015 in Berlin by M Kunze et al. on vaginal and vagino-rectal samples taken pre-partum between 35 and 37 weeks' gestation. Intrapartum samples were exclusively vaginorectal with a prevalence of maternal GBS colonisation of 17% (11).

Bassir A et al (6) published in 2016 their study carried out in Morocco in the Marrakech region with a GBS carriage prevalence of 20.2% on vaginal samples.

Moraleda C et al (15) put the prevalence of GBS carriage in pregnant women between 34 and 37 years of age in the Rabat region in 2017 at 24% on vaginal-rectal swabs.

In Tunisia, Skhiri I, based on vaginal swabs, found a prevalence of 7.3% in a study carried out in 2010 in the Monastir region (7).

II. Factors influencing prevalence

Variability in the prevalence of GBS carriage depends on the sampling site, the population studied, the culture medium used and the screening term.

1. Screening term

Rectal and vaginal colonisation with streptococcus B may be persistent, transient or intermittent. Some authors believe that virtually all pregnant women are colonised at some point during pregnancy (17). The relationship between carriage during pregnancy and carriage at delivery is unpredictable (18).

According to a series by Valkenburg-van den Berget al published in 2010, the positive predictive value decreases when the interval between prenatal and delivery cultures increases, particularly when it exceeds 6 weeks. In addition, it is possible that women whose screening was negative in early pregnancy may have contracted GBS later, as GBS colonisation is not constant. For this reason, the Centers for Disease Control and Prevention (CDCP) strongly recommends the collection of recto-vaginal cultures during the 35-37 SA antenatal period (19).

Although vaginal carriage is very inconstant during pregnancy, Boyer showed that all parturients who had a PV (+) less than 6 weeks before delivery had it during labour (20).

2. Sampling site

Streptococcus B colonises the genital region more than the vaginal canal. The most appropriate site for sampling is the distal part of the vagina without reaching the cervix and genital area (21,22).

Sampling the vaginal and rectal regions gives a significantly higher percentage of GBS colonisation, as vaginal or cervical samples are not optimal and lead to a 40% reduction in positive results. Although perianal swabs may be equivalent to rectal swabs, collection of this sample may not be adequate in the general population and has not been formally approved (23).

In 2011, the ACOG reiterated the importance of collecting vaginal and rectal swabs (from the lower vagina and then through the anal canal)(24).

Meyn et al. believe that the prevalence of GBS colonisation is due to rectal rather than vaginal colonisation and that rectal location is the only determinant of vaginal location (25).

III. RISK FACTORS FOR MATERNAL COLONISATION Risk factors for maternal colonisation

Many studies have focused on GBS and its microbiological properties, but few have identified the risk factors for maternal carriage.

In Algeria, a study carried out in 2017 found a prevalence of vaginal GBS carriage of 22.6% and found no risk factors related to obstetric antecedents favouring vaginal GBS carriage (16).

In 2015 Cools P et al identified risk factors for GBS carriage, namely recent sexual intercourse, douching for hygienic purposes, colonisation with Candida Albicans and the presence of a cervical ectropion. Women were twice as likely to be colonised by GBS when they washed inside the vagina with a substance other than water, such as water mixed with vinegar or antiseptic products, a common practice in Africa, than women who did not wash inside the vagina. They also hypothesised that sexual activity during pregnancy could lead to a brief temporal colonisation of the vagina by GBS. However, their results did not reach significance, probably due to the small sample size (26).

As for Mitima et al., maternal colonisation by GBS is 20% in DR Congo and is significantly associated with a low level of education, genitourinary tract infections during pregnancy, HIV infection and a history of abortion and/or premature delivery (10).

Socio-economic status can be indirectly reflected by education level and employment status. Lack of education has been identified as a risk factor for GBS colonisation, whereas unemployment has not (13,27).

Arain F R et al found in Saudi Arabia that maternal colonisation by GBS was significantly associated with the type of work done by women, with housewives and doctors having a very significant incidence. Neither primiparity nor multiparity was associated with maternal colonisation (12).

A South African study of 340 women showed that history of stillbirth, miscarriage, lack of education and HIV(+) serology were risk factors for maternal carriage of GBS (13).

In an adjusted analysis carried out in The Gambia in 2015, maternal haemoglobin <10 g/dL and a history of more than one stillbirth were associated with increased risk of GBS colonisation by the mother at delivery (14).

In Marrakech, a 2016 study found no risk factors associated with maternal carriage of GBS. Age, parity, gestational age and gynaecological and obstetric antecedents had no influence (6).

A study published in 2009 in the UK found that newborn GBS infection was strongly associated with chronic maternal GBS carriage (28).

Neither gestational age and parity nor a history of spontaneous miscarriage (SCF) or diabetes were considered as risk factors associated with GBS in the study conducted by M.UDAHEMUKA (29).

In Tunisia, Skhiri I studied the risk factors for maternal GBS carriage in 2010 and identified a significant association between GBS carriage and low level of education, previous history of SCF and gestational diabetes (7).

In our adjusted study, the risk factors for vaginal carriage of GBS were rural residence and a history of diabetes. History of

porting of the SGB was significant but eliminated after binary logistic regression.

A cause and effect relationship could not be established between gestational diabetes and GBS; the difference between the two groups was not significant (p=0.181).

IV. Vaginal carriage and the course of pregnancy

Various series in the literature have studied the effect of carriage of group B Streptococcus on the course of pregnancy and its consequences for childbirth.

1. MFIU

According to a meta-analysis carried out in 2017 in different continents and regions of the world, A C. Seale et al. Seale et al. estimate that GBS is likely to account for more MFIU than neonatal death.

Seale et al. estimate that 1% of all UFIDs in developed countries and 4% in Africa are associated with GBS (30).

Two UK studies concluded that GBS disease in pregnant women is strongly associated with pre- and post-natal mortality (31,32).

According to a study carried out in Kenya in 2016, GBS is an important, potentially preventable, cause of IUGR and neonatal death. Even so, the incidences found are all underestimated(33).

According to a study in Reunion, perinatal infections were the leading cause of UFI (26.4% of cases), with streptococcus B being the most frequent germ (34).

In our series, eight MFIU were noted. However, a causal relationship could not be established. The difference between the two groups was statistically insignificant.

2. RPM, prematurity and IUGR

Heath P T et al reported that premature rupture of membranes was an important factor associated with GBS infection of the newborn. Prematurity was associated with GBS but did not reach significance (28).

A meta-analysis by Bianchi-jassir et al. published in 2017, which included 45 studies, most of which were from developed countries, including 8 from the United States and 22 from Europe, found a clear association between GBS and premature birth. Thus there was evidence of an association between maternal GBS colonisation and prematurity in cohort and cross-sectional studies (hazard ratio [HR], 1.21 [95% confidence interval {CI}, .99-1.48]; P = 0.061) and in case-control studies (odds ratio [OR], 1.85 [95% CI, 1.24 to 2.77]; P = 0.003) (35).

M.UDAHEMUKA in his study carried out in Rabat in 2013 did not link streptococcus B to the occurrence of PAD during pregnancy (29).

In a Korean study, Kim et al. did not identify any factors associated with GBS, but PMR of 18 hours or more was associated with a high prevalence of GBS colonisation, but not significantly (p=0.079) (36).

A study published in 2014 reported that GBS bacteriuria, prematurity <37 SA and PMR >18h were risk factors associated with neonatal GBS infection (23).

For Hornik, IUGR is strongly associated with GBS (37).

Other studies have found no correlation between intrauterine growth retardation and streptococcus B (13,38).

In our series :

• IUGR was statistically associated with carriage of group B streptococcus but was not significant in multivariate regression (p=0.046).

• No statistically significant correlation was found between prematurity and streptococcus B carriage (p=0.577).

• Pre-term MTR after screening was noted in 17 patients, including one with GBS. The difference between the two groups was not significant.

V. Factor in maternal-fetal transmission

Since the 1970s, the incidence of group B streptococcal septicaemia and neonatal meningitis has risen considerably in all industrialised countries. They affect between 0.5 and 1% of newborns in developed countries and 3 to 5% in developing countries, with a mortality rate of around 20% (16). Early-onset neonatal bacterial infection (EBNI) is almost exclusively due to maternal-fetal transmission. Transmission occurs by the ascending route or during passage through the vaginal tract, and very rarely by the hematogenic route (3).

Le Doare et al found that the presence at delivery of a midwife rather than a skilled birth attendant and delivery during the wet season or dry heat were associated with an increased risk of GBS colonisation by the mother during delivery (14).

Dahan-Saal,J et al. have demonstrated the protective role of cesarean section and intrapartum antibiotic prophylaxis (IPP) in the vertical transmission of GBS. Maternal obesity and late prematurity are not considered to be determining factors per se, but rather to favour GBS transmission (39).

In the UK, Heath et al found a highly significant association between GBS infection of the newborn and maternal intrapartum fever (28).

Intrapartum maternal fever (temperature >38°) was considered to be a risk factor associated with neonatal GBS infection (23,40).

In our study, no factor was significantly associated with GBS carriage. None of the patients in the streptococcus B+ group developed an intrapartum fever (p=0.917).

VI. New colonised mother

1. Apgar

The Apgar problem has received little attention in the various series published in the literature.

The mean Apgar score at five minutes for Jerbi et al. was 9.73, with a non-significant difference (p=0.8) (41).

Similarly, in 2010, Skhiri found no significant difference between the babies of treated mothers and those of untreated mothers.

2. Newborn infection

2.1. Incidence of GBS MFIs

The overall incidence varies from 0.2 to 10 per 1000 live births, depending on the country and whether or not probable infections are taken into account(42).

Table XVI: GBS infection rates per live birth according to the literature

Country	Year	Incidence of infection
United States (43)	1990	1.7 %%
North Carolina/ United States (44)	1997-2001	3.5 %
United States(43)	2000	0.25 %
North Carolina/ United States (44)	2002-2010	2.6 %
United Kingdom (45)	2004-2007	0.52 %
France (46)	2005	8.15 %
England (47)	2006-2008	0.9 %

In the study carried out by Muris et al. based on Anaes recommendations, the protocol proved effective in reducing the number of maternal-fctal infections, without increasing the number of infections with germs other than GBS, and without increasing the number of children hospitalised for suspected infection (40). The GBS mortality rate fell from 20-50% in 1999 to 5% in 2005 in the United States (48).

2.2. Neonatal care

According to the CDC's recommendations, revised in 2010, the management of newborn infants of carrier-positive mothers who have received antibiotic prophylaxis includes (49):

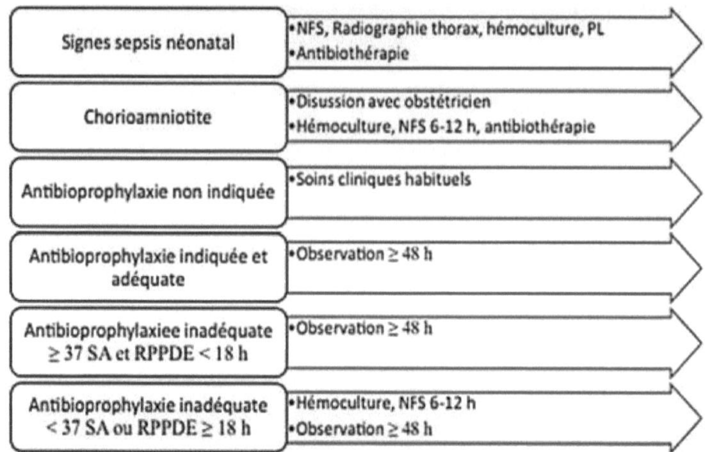

Figure 1: Algorithm for the management of newborn babies (49).

The COFN has suggested a number of variants to this algorithm (50) :

• The indications for lumbar puncture (LP) have been clarified. If the obstetric history does not identify any risk factors for sepsis, a period of 4 to 6 hours' observation is permitted. LP is still indicated if the blood culture (HC) is positive, if the biological data are suggestive of bacterial infection, and in neonates who do not respond to conventional antibiotic therapy;

• in the case of inadequate IPA in an asymptomatic child (excluding chorioamniotitis):

J Prolonged rupture of the water sac (RPPDE) < 18 h: clinical monitoring has been extended to 35-36 SA,

J RPPDE 18 h and > 37 SA: clinical monitoring was recommended,

J prematurity <37 SA: blood culture not necessary (unless antibiotic therapy is decided), CRP at 6-12 h possible.

The main changes in the new recommendations of the Haute Autorite de Sante (HAS) 2017(51)

• The use of TBAs in asymptomatic newborns should be the exception rather than the rule.

• Early detection of signs of infection is essential to avoid delaying the initiation of antibiotic therapy, given the known adverse consequences on morbidity and mortality.

• Standardised clinical monitoring in maternity wards should be preferred to probabilistic antibiotic therapy in asymptomatic infants. Training and support for healthcare teams in the implementation of such monitoring is essential to its success and effectiveness.

• The role of CRP and PCT measured in cord blood and postnatally in the initiation, discontinuation and monitoring of TBA should be clarified in the near future and supplement the HAS 2017 recommendations.

In our series, neonatal management did not depend on the number of doses received by the mother, but we have :

• Performs peripheral swabs on newborns born to mothers with GBS who have given birth vaginally (4 hospitalised and 5 non-hospitalised newborns benefited from these tests)

• Carry out a CRP test at H12 and H24 on all newborns of positive mothers.

• Monitor all newborns for at least 24 hours.

• Provision for central sampling in the event of the appearance of clinical signs, whether or not associated with biological disturbances.

VII. Screening and diagnostic strategy

1. Diagnosis+ prenatal; For whom

1.1. According to Royal College of Obstetricians and Gynaecologists (RCOG) 2017 United-Kingdom (UK).

The National Screening Committee does not recommend universal bacteriological screening for GBS. Their view is that there is no clear evidence to demonstrate that GBS screening would systematically do more good than harm. The reasons cited are:

• Many women are carriers of the bacterium and, in the majority of cases, their babies are born safely and without developing an infection.

• Screening women in late pregnancy cannot accurately predict which babies will develop GBS infection.

• No screening test is completely accurate. Between 17% and 25% of women who have a positive vaginal smear between 35 and 37 weeks' gestation will be GBS-negative at delivery. Between 5% and 7% of women who are GBS-negative between 35 and 37 weeks' gestation will be GBS-negative at the time of delivery.

• In addition, many babies with severe GBS infection are born prematurely, before the suggested screening time.

• Giving all GBS carriers an AIP would mean that a very large number of women would receive treatment that they did not need; this may increase the harmful consequences for both mother and baby.

This is why GBS screening of all pregnant women is not routinely offered in the UK (52).

1.2. According to the Council of the Society of Obstetricians and Gynaecologists of Canada 2018

Offer all women screening for group B streptococcal colonisation at 35 - 37 weeks' gestation by means of culture from a swab of the vagina first and then the rectum (beyond the anal sphincter). (II-1A) This approach also applies to women who are scheduled for caesarean section because of their risk of labour or rupture of membranes before the scheduled date of caesarean section (53).

2. Microbiological diagnostic methods

France 2014

In France, several selective or chromogenic media for the isolation and identification of S. Agalactie are marketed, making antenatal screening easier. Rapid diagnostic tests based on immunology or molecular biology techniques are also available for hospitalized pregnant women who have not been able to benefit from prior screening (premature rupture of membranes, threat of premature delivery, lack of medical follow-up, etc.). The StrepB OIAW immuno-optical device, based on recognition of specific S. agalactie antigens from biological samples, provides a result in less than 30 minutes, but lacks sensitivity. Molecular biology techniques, in particular Polymerase Chain Reaction (PCR), on the other hand, have excellent sensitivity and specificity, and the availability of commercial kits and automated systems means that they can now be used at the patient's bedside. In the USA and Canada, these techniques are recommended for full-term women with unknown carriage status (54).

United Kingdom 2017

Enriched culture media tests are recommended. The clinician should indicate that the swab is taken for GBS.

Polymerase chain reaction or any other screening test carried out near the patient in early labour is not recommended.

The evidence does not suggest that the use of polymerase chain reaction technology for near-patient testing is feasible in UK maternity services. Near-patient testing technology continues to improve and it is possible that this will confer benefits in the future.

Canada 2018

The 2010 CDC guideline states that a useful intrapartum screening test should be simple, have a turnaround time of <30 minutes and have a sensitivity and specificity of 90%. This technique would be reserved for hospitals with a diagnostic laboratory capable of real-time PCR screening, valid PCR performance and adequate quality control measures. A study comparing intrapartum screening for early-onset GBS infection by PCR (Xpert GBS test) with prenatal screening by culture of a swab taken from the lower vagina, in terms of estimated direct costs and outcomes (including costs associated with screening and hospitalisation), found that PCR was associated with an increased detection rate of GBS colonisation (16.7% vs 11.7%).

Thanks to improved techniques, GBS screening could be replaced by intrapartum PCR screening in some institutions (53).

3. Therapeutic management and antibiotic prophylaxis

3.1. Indications

Canada 2018

Because of the association between heavy colonisation and early-onset neonatal infection, administer intravenous antibiotic prophylaxis against group B streptococci in the following cases, at the time of onset of labour or rupture of membranes:

• all women with positive results (indicating the presence of group B streptococci) in the culture-based screening of a vaginal/rectal swab taken at 35 - 37 weeks' gestation (II-2B);

• any woman who has already given birth to a child with group B streptococcal infection (II-3B);

• any woman with documented group B streptococcal bacteriuria (regardless of colony-forming unit count) in the current pregnancy. (II-2A)

Administer intravenous antibiotic prophylaxis for group B streptococci for a minimum of 48 hours to all women < 37 weeks gestation with labour or rupture of membranes, except where a negative result has been obtained in the preceding five weeks by a rapid nucleic acid-based test or vaginal/rectal swab culture screening (II-3A).

Administer (intravenously) broad-spectrum antibiotics targeting chorioamniotitis and group B streptococci to all women presenting with intrapartum fever and symptoms of chorioamniotitis (regardless of gestational age or group B streptococcal status).

UK 2017

Prenatal treatment for vaginal or rectal colonisation does not reduce the risk of GBS colonisation at the time of delivery and is therefore not indicated prior to the onset of labour. AIP should be indicated for women colonised with GBS.

GBS bacteriuria is associated with a higher risk of chorioamniotitis and neonatal disease, although it is not possible to quantify these risks accurately. Women with GBS bacteriuria should be offered anti-infective treatment. Women with GBS urinary tract infection during pregnancy (growth greater than 10*5 cfu / ml) should receive appropriate treatment at the time of diagnosis and intrapartum.

Women presenting with a fever >38C should be given a broad-spectrum IPB covering GBS, to be adapted according to the results of the antibiogram.

Women who are not known to be GBS carriers and who go into preterm labour should be treated with IAP. This antibiotic treatment is not recommended for women who are not in labour and who have a scheduled caesarean section with intact membranes.

3.2. Therapeutic means

Canada 2018

1. Penicillin G (Peni G), 5 million units IV, then 2.5 to 3.0 million every 4 hours, until delivery or

2. When the patient is allergic to penicillin, but is exposed to only a low risk of anaphylaxis: cefazolin, 2 g IV, then 1 g every 8 hours until delivery or

3. When the patient is allergic to penicillin and at risk of anaphylaxis: clindamycin, 900 mg IV every 8 hours until delivery (when the isolate is sensitive to clindamycin without inducible resistance), or vancomycin, 1 g IV every 12 hours until delivery.

UK 2017

For women in whom DPI has been indicated, benzylpenicillin should be administered. Once started, treatment should be administered regularly until delivery.

It is recommended that 3g of benzylpenicillin be administered intravenously as soon as possible after the onset of labour and 1.5g every 4 hours until delivery. To optimise the efficacy of IAP, the first dose should be administered at least 4 hours before delivery.

If the history is suggestive of allergy to beta-lactams, but not severe (i.e. no anaphylaxis, angioedema, respiratory distress (RD) or urticaria), an intravenous cephalosporin can be administered (cefuroxime, loading dose of 1.5g followed by 750mg 8 hours). If the allergy to beta-lactams is severe, intravenous vancomycin (1g every 12 hours) is recommended.

4. Revised recommendations

The widespread implementation of GBS infection prevention programmes since the early 2000s has made it possible to analyse their effectiveness and identify the risks of antibiotic treatment prescribed to almost 30% of pregnant women and 2-10% of newborns(55). These considerations led to changes in the recommendations from 2010 onwards.

4.1. In the United Kingdom (RCOG)

In July 2012, the RCOG published an update of its recommendations. Systematic screening for GBS carriage was still not recommended.

This position was justified by the low rate of early neonatal infection in the United Kingdom (0.50/1000), which is close to that in the United States after the implementation of systematic screening, and by the conclusions of a Cochrane review which showed no proven effect on reducing GBS-related mortality (56). With regard to neonatal management, the RCOG only requires immediate antibiotic treatment in the presence of clinical signs of NPI. In other situations, a 24-hour period of clinical observation is suggested, without any additional biological tests (57).

4.2. Recommendations from the CDC, the American Academy of Pediatrics (AAP) and the Committee on Fetus and Newborn (COFN)

In 2010, the CDC published revised recommendations approved by the AAP and the COFN in 2011(49,58). In 2012, the COFN published recommendations on the management of newborns with suspected or proven NPI, specifying the indications for biological evaluation and the duration of antibiotic therapy (59). In 2013, Polin, the first author of this text, clarified the COFN's position due to discrepancies in the management algorithms between the CDC's 2010 recommendations and those of the COFN in 2012 (50).

With regard to primary prevention in pregnant women, the main changes concern :

• description of antibiotic-supplemented selective culture media or chromogenic media to be used for antenatal screening for GBS in order to increase sensitivity;

• the possibility of using rapid GBS screening tests by polymerase chain reaction (PCR) intrapartum, reserving them for situations where GBS colonisation is not known at term;

• precision of the algorithm for indications of AIP in cases of threatened premature delivery and preterm PMR; antibiotic therapy in penicillin-allergic patients: cefazolin in cases of low anaphylactic risk, clindamycin or vancomycin in cases of high anaphylactic risk according to the antibiogram;

• 1 adequate AIP defined as at least 4 hours of penicillin, ampicillin or cefazolin.

VIII. Limitations of the study

During the course of our work, we were confronted with a number of factors that limited our study:

- The absence of a rectal swab combined with a vaginal swab.

- No use of a non-nutritive transport medium.

- The use of an enriched and selective medium, admittedly, but as recommended (we did not use the Todd-Hewitt medium).

- The target population: the patients screened in our series were those who had visited the maternity hospital for one reason or another during the third trimester, which made the sample unrepresentative, creating a selection bias that led to an underestimation of the rate.

- A not insignificant number of women who have had a PV carried out have been lost to follow-up.

- The small number of GBS-colonised pregnant patients screened during this period.

As our results are based on an observational rather than an experimental study design, they could be explained by factors other than the screening programme.

IX. Perspective

1. Vaginal disinfection

In view of the results of the various studies carried out on the seriousness of GBS infection in newborns and parturients, it seems relatively important to continue to raise awareness among healthcare professionals of the importance of a well-conducted screening policy.

Low frequency of daily hand washing by the nursing staff was associated with maternal colonisation with GBS (60).

A study by Foxman B et al. found no significant association between GBS carriage and handwashing practices, although there was a downward trend in incidence with increased frequency of handwashing for capsular type V and all capsular types combined (61).

Information aimed at potential samplers on the conditions under which a vaginal sample should be taken as part of GBS screening should be considered (62).

Hygiene conditions must be observed, and hands must be washed in a hospital or rubbed with a hydro-alcoholic solution prior to the procedure (62).

2. Vaccination

The increasing incidence of Streptococcus B infections in adults and the ineffectiveness of antibiotic prophylaxis in reducing late neonatal infections demonstrate the importance of developing new means of prevention.

One preferred approach is vaccination, which would prevent infections in adults as well as neonatal infections by transmitting maternal antibodies to the newborn.

GBS surface proteins have also been studied as potential vaccine components. An immunogenic surface protein conserved in all strains of Streptococcus B would make an ideal vaccine target. In addition, the reverse vaccinology strategy based on the identification of vaccine targets by genomic analysis, already applied for Neisseria meningitidis serotype B, was used for GBS. Candidate proteins are identified, produced and then tested in animal models. Several vaccine targets have been selected (the secreted protein Sip and three pili components) but, to date, this approach has not led to the identification of a universal antigen (54).

According to the World Health Organization (WHO) 2017, there is currently no preventive vaccine against GBS, but maternal immunisation with several serotypes of protein-conjugated anti-GBS capsular polysaccharides may reduce the risk of disease in newborns and young children through trans-placental passage of protective immunoglobulins. Candidate protein-based vaccines are also being evaluated (63).

The potential impact of the introduction of the vaccine on the use of perinatal antibiotics is a critical aspect that needs to be assessed in view of the global problem of antimicrobial resistance and emerging data on the importance of preserving the neonatal microbiome (63).

CONCLUSION

Group B Streptococcus, or Streptococcus Agalactiae, has been identified as the main cause of invasive bacterial infections in newborn babies.

This bacterium intermittently colonises the vaginal cavity of several women, who are considered to be "healthy" carriers.

Transmission occurs via the ascending route or when passing through the vaginal birth canal, and very rarely via hematogenesis.

The prevalence of GBS carriage worldwide is estimated at 18%, with an average ranging from 11% to 35%.

Recommendations have been put forward, with the superiority of the strategy based on systematic screening of all pregnant women, ideally between 35 and 37 weeks' amenorrhoea, followed by prophylactic intrapartum antibiotic treatment for colonised women.

Even perfect adherence to the recommended prevention guidelines would not allow complete prevention of neonatal GBS infection, which is why we proposed to evaluate the proportion of streptococcus B in daily practice in our maternity hospital through a cross-sectional study with the aim of :

- To determine the prevalence of vaginal carriage of streptococcus B in the third trimester of pregnancy.

- Identify the main risk factors for portage.

- Defining a screening strategy for streptococcus B.

- To determine the diagnostic and therapeutic means of vaginal carriage of GBS.

A cross-sectional study was carried out in the obstetric gynaecology department of Monastir University Hospital, including 330 women in their third trimester who were screened from 34 weeks' gestation.

Patients were excluded from the study:

- Clinical signs (leucorrhoea; uterine contractions; PNAg or RPM)

- I had received antibiotics 15 days previously.

We tested for streptococcus B by taking a vaginal swab at the antenatal clinic between 34 and 38 weeks' gestation.

In accordance with ANAES recommendations published in September 2001, the vaginal swab was taken in the examination room, with the parturient in the gynaecological position, using a swab without a speculum, sweeping the lower third of the vagina as far as the vestibule and vulva, without reaching the posterior vaginal pouch and without taking an associated rectal swab.

The sample was delivered rapidly to the bacteriology laboratory, without any preservation medium, within half an hour.

Patients labelled as streptococcus B positive were given appropriate intravenous antibiotic therapy from the onset of labour, and their newborn infants were monitored clinically with peripheral samples and CRP kinetics.

The carry rate in our series was **8.8%.**

More than half of the women were of urban origin. A history of diabetes was noted in 8.2% of cases. Primiparity was noted in 35.5% of cases. FCS was predominant in 73 patients, i.e. 22.1% of cases. Sixteen patients had multiple pregnancies, two of which were triplets.

Gestational diabetes was noted in 27.9% of cases. 5.2% of women had preterm PPROM after PV, 51 IUGR (15.6% of cases). Prematurity was noted in 24% of cases. 8 cases of MFIU were noted, i.e. 2.4% of cases.

The molecule of choice for antibiotic prophylaxis was Totapen in 77.22% of cases. In cases of allergy, a macrolide was used.

Four newborn babies born to mothers carrying streptococcus B were admitted to hospital.

The factors associated with streptococcus B carriage were :
- Rural origin (p=0.027).
- History of diabetes $(p<10)^{-3}$
- Previous streptococcus B carriage (p=0.007).
- IUGR (p=0.046).

The risk factors for streptococcus B carriage were :
- living in rural areas OR = 2.7; CI [1.084 -6.764], p=0.033
- history of diabetes OR = 27.6; CI [10.498-72.536], $p<10 .^{-3}$

MFI is common. The morbidity and mortality associated with it reflect its seriousness, despite advances in management. It is therefore necessary to increase efforts in antenatal prevention and to make antibiotic treatment decisions for newborns with suspected infection adapted to the microbial epidemiology (64).

The screening protocol must be drawn up by a multidisciplinary team involving obstetricians, midwives, neonatologists and bacteriologists.

Rational multicentre studies, such as the one carried out in the United Kingdom(57) and the one by Neal j Russel et al.(4), could give a more precise idea of the frequency of carriage and the methods for setting up and applying a screening protocol.

Antigenic techniques for rapid detection of this type of carriage may be useful in certain cases, provided they are validated and their cost is taken into account.

The trend in recent recommendations is to limit the need for additional investigations and probabilistic antibiotic therapy in low-risk situations, in favour of close clinical monitoring. The separation of mother and child, the risk of antibiotic resistance developing, iatrogenic complications during hospitalisation and the long-term consequences of antibiotic treatment in the first few days of life due to changes in the macrobiota justify this approach.

Nevertheless, even perfect adherence to the recommended prevention guidelines would not completely prevent neonatal GBS infection and, despite the efforts made, a significant proportion of permanent neurological sequelae and mortality would still occur. Vaccination of pregnant women is an important and desirable strategy to ensure that levels of protection are maintained.

A trivalent conjugate vaccine (serotypes Ia, Ib and III) is currently being tested in healthy pregnant women; this will eventually reduce not only the burden of early neonatal infection (ENI), but also that of GBS-related premature births and late neonatal infection.

In view of the above, this pre-vaccine era emphasises the importance of maintaining surveillance systems to monitor the impact of future vaccines and to support effective strategies to prevent GBS disease in newborns (65).

BIBLIOGRAPHY

1. Quentin R, Morange-Saussier V, Watt S. Management of Streptococcus agalactiae in obstetrics. J Gynecol Obstet Biol Reprod. 2008; 31 (Suppl 6):65-73.

2. Assouik F,Z. Vaginal carriage of group B Streptococcus in women. http://ao.um5s.ac.ma/xmlui/handle/123456789/361, accessed 13 July 2019

3. Thibaudon Baveux C, Stroebel Noguer A, Boulard Mallet I, Djavadzadeh-Amini M, Kacet N, Truffert P, et al. Prevention des infections bacteriennes neonatales precoces a streptocoque B. J Gynecol Obstet Biol Reprod. 2008;37(4):392-9.

4. Russell N J, Seale A C, O'Driscoll M, O'Sullivan C, Bianchi-Jassir F, Maternal Colonization With Group B Streptococcus and Serotype Distribution Worldwide: Systematic Review and Meta-analyses. Clin Infect Dis. 2017; 65 (suppl 2): S100-S111.

5. Chhuy T, Mansour G, Zejli A, Bouquigny C, Bock S, Abboud P, Depistage du streptocoque de groupe B pendant la grossesse: A propos de 1 674 prelevements. J Gynecol Obstet Biol Reprod. 2005;34 (4): 328-33.

6. Bassir A, Dhibou H, Farah M, Mohamed L, Amal A, Nabila S, et al. Vaginal carriage of group B streptococcus in pregnant women in the Marrakech region. Pan Afr Med J.2016;23:107.

7. Skhiri Ep Bouzguenda I. Screening for group B streptococcus in pregnant women in the third trimester. Th D Med, Monastir; 2010.

8. Kwatra G, Adrian PV, Shiri T, Buchmann EJ, Cutland CL, et al. SerotypeSpecific Acquisition and Loss of Group B Streptococcus Recto-Vaginal Colonization in Late Pregnancy. Plos One. 2014; 9(6):e98778.

9. Shirazi M, Abbariki E, Hafizi A, Shahbazi F, Bandari M, Dastgerdy E. The Prevalence of Group B Streptococcus Colonization in Iranian Pregnant Women and Its Subsequent Outcome. Int J Fertil Steril. 2014;7(4):267-70.

10. Mitima KT, Ntamako S, Birindwa AM, Mukanire N, Kivukuto JM, Tsongo K, et al. Prevalence of colonization by Streptococcus agalactiae among pregnant

women in Bukavu, Democratic Republic of the Congo. J Infect Dev Ctries. 2014;8(09):1195-200.

11. Kunze M, Zumstein K, Markfeld-Erol F, Elling R, Lander F, Prompeler H, et al. Comparison of pre- and intrapartum screening of group B streptococci and adherence to screening guidelines: a cohort study. Eur J Pediatr.2015;174(6):827-35.

12. Arain FR, Al-Bezrah NA, Al-Aali KY. Prevalence of Maternal Genital Tract Colonization by Group B Streptococcus From Western Province, Taif, Saudi Arabia. J Clin Gynecol Obstet. 2015;4(3):258-264-264.

13. Matsiane Lekala L. Risk Factors Associated with Group B Streptococcus Colonization and Their Effect on Pregnancy Outcome. J Gynecol Obstet. 2015;3(6):121.

14. Le Doare K, Jarju S, Darboe S, Warburton F, Gorringe A, Heath PT, et al. Risk factors for Group B Streptococcus colonisation and disease in Gambian women and their infants. J Infect. 2016;72(3):283-94.

15. Moraleda C, Ben Messaoud R, Esteban J, Lopez Y.Prevalence, antimicrobial resistance and serotype distribution of group B streptococcus isolated among pregnant women and newborns in Rabat, Morocco. J Med Microbiol. 2018.doi:10.1099/jmm.0.000720.[Epub a Read of print].

16. Mahrane ep Bouchenou S. Infections maternofoetales a Streptococcus agalactiae: Etude du portage chez la femme enceinte, des infections neonatales et caracterisation des souches invasives. Th D Med, Alger; 2017.

17. Gibbs RS, Schrag S, Schuchat A. Perinatal Infections Due to Group B Streptococci: Obstet Gynecol. 2004;104(5, Part 1):1062-76.

18. Honderlick P, Gravisse J, Cahen P, Vignou D. Bacteriological assessment of six years of group B streptococcus (GBS) screening in the last trimester of pregnancy. Pathol Biol. 2010; 58(2):144-6.

19. Valkenburg-van den Berg AW, Houtman-Roelofsen RL, Oostvogel PM, Dekker FW, Dorr PJ, Sprij AJ. Timing of Group B Streptococcus Screening in Pregnancy: A Systematic Review. Gynecol Obstet Invest. 2010;69(3):174-83.

20. Boyer KM, Gadzala CA, Kelly PD, Burd LI, Gotoff SP. Selective Intrapartum Chemoprophylaxis of Neonatal Group B Streptococcal Early- Onset Disease. II. Predictive Value of Prenatal Cultures. J Infect Dis. 1983;148(5):802-9.

21. Larsen JW, Sever JL. Group B Streptococcus and pregnancy: a review. Am J Obstet Gynecol. 2008;198(4):440-50.

22. El Beitune P, Duarte G, Maffei CML, Quintana SM, De Sa Rosa E Silva ACJ, Nogueira AA. Group B Streptococcus carriers among HIV-1 infected pregnant women: Prevalence and risk factors. Eur J Obstet Gynecol Reprod Biol. 2006;128(1):54-8.

23. Ahmadzia HK, Heine RP. Diagnosis and Management of Group B Streptococcus in Pregnancy. Obstet Gynecol Clin. 2014;41(4):629-47.

24. American College of Obstetricians and Gynecologists. ACOG Committee Opinion: number 279, December 2002. Prevention of early-onset group B streptococcal disease in newborns. Obstet Gynecol. 2002;100(6):1405-12.

25. Meyn LA, Krohn MA, Hillier SL. Rectal colonization by group B Streptococcus as a predictor of vaginal colonization. Am J Obstet Gynecol. 2009;201(1):76.e1-7.

26. Cools P, Jespers V, Hardy L, Grucitti T,. A Multi-Country Cross-Sectional Study of Vaginal Carriage of Group B Streptococci (GBS) and Escherichia coli in Resource-Poor Settings: Prevalences and Risk Factors. Plos One. 2016;11(1): eO148052.

27. Tsolia M, Psoma M, Gavrili S, Petrochilou V, Michalas S, Legakis N, et al. Group B streptococcus colonization of Greek pregnant women and neonates: prevalence, risk factors and serotypes. Clin Microbiol Infect. 2003;9(8):832-8.

28. Heath PT, Balfour GF, Tighe H, Verlander NQ, Lamagni TL, Efstratiou A, et al. Group B streptococcal disease in infants: a case control study. Arch Dis Child. 2009;94(9):674-80.

29. Marguerite U. Prevalence of streptococcus B in pregnant women attending l'hopital militaire d'instruction mohamed 5 a rabat.

http://ao.um5s.aac.ma/xmlui/handle/123456789/946. accessed 14 July 2019.

30. Seale AC, Blencowe H, Bianchi-Jassir F, Embleton N, Bassat Q, Ordi J, et al. Stillbirth With Group B Streptococcus Disease Worldwide: Systematic Review and Meta-analyses. Clin Infect Dis. 2017;65(suppl 2):S125-32.

31. Kalin A, Acosta C, Kurinzuk JJ. Severe sepsis in women with group B Streptococcus in pregnancy: an exploratory UK national case-control study. BMJO pen. 2015;5(10):e007976.

32. Deutscher M, Lewis M, Zell ER, Taylor THJr. Incidence and Severity of Invasive Streptococcus pneumoniae, Group A Streptococcus, and Group B Streptococcus Infections Among Pregnant and Postpartum Women. Clin Infect Dis. 2011;53(2):114-23.

33. Seale AC, Koech AC, Sheppard AE, Barsosio HC, Langat J, Anyango E, et al. Maternal colonization with *Streptococcus agalactiae* and associated stillbirth and neonatal disease in coastal Kenya. Nat Microbiol. 2016;1(7):16067.

34. Andriamandimbison Z, Randriambololona DMA, Rasoanandrianina BS, Hery RA. Causes of in utero fetal deaths: 225 cases at Befelatanana Hospital, Madagascar. Medecine Sante Trop. 2013;23(1):78-82.

35. Bianchi-Jassir F, Seale AC, Kohli-Lynch M, Lawn JE, Baker CJ, Bartlett L, et al. Preterm Birth Associated With Group B Streptococcus Maternal Colonization Worldwide: Systematic Review and Meta-analyses. Clin Infect Dis. 2017;65(suppl_2):S133-42.

36. Kim EJ, Oh KY, Kim MY, Seo YS, Shin J-H, Song YR, et al. Risk Factors for Group B Streptococcus Colonization Among Pregnant Women in Korea. Epidemiol Health. 2011;33:e2011010.

37. Hornik CP, Fort P, Clark RH, Watt K, Benjamin DK, Smith PB, et al. Early and late onset sepsis in very-low-birth-weight infants from a large group of neonatal intensive care units. Early Hum Dev. 2012;88:S69-74.

38. Klinger G, Levy I, Sirota L, Boyko V, Reichman B, Lerner-Geva L. Epidemiology and risk factors for early onset sepsis among very-low-birthweight infants. Am J Obstet Gynecol. 2009;201(1):38.e1-38.e6.

39. Dahan-Saal J, Gerardin P, Robillard P-Y, Barau G, Bouveret A, Picot S, et al. Determinants of maternal streptococcal B colonisation and factors associated with its perinatal vertical transmission: a case-control study. Gynecol Obstet Fertil. 2011;39(5):281-8.

40. Muris C, Lemonnier M, Herlicoviez M, Dreyfus M. Prevention des infections maternofctales a streptocoque B. 1. Application des recommandations de l'Anaes. J Gynecol Obstet Biol Reprod. 2010;39(7):554-9.

41. Jerbi M, Hidar S, Hannachi N, El Moueddeb S, Djebbari H, Boukadida J, et al. Risk factors for carriage of group B streptococcus in pregnant women at term: a prospective study of 294 cases. Gynecol Obstet Fertil. 2007;35(4):312-6.

42. Nizet V, Klein JO. Bacterial sepsis and meningitis. Infect Dis Fetus Newborn. 2011;7:223-64.

43. Hyde TB, Hilger TM, Reingold A, Farley MM. Trends in Incidence and Antimicrobial Resistance of Early-Onset Sepsis: Population-Based Surveillance in San Francisco and Atlanta. Pediatrics. 2002;110(4):690-5.

44. Bauserman MS, Laughon MM, Hornik CP, Smith PB, Benjamin DK, Clark RH, et al. Group B Streptococcus and Escherichia coli Infections in the Intensive Care Nursery in the Era of Intrapartum Antibiotic Prophylaxis. Pediatr Infect Dis J. 2013;32(3):208-12.

45. Vergnano S, Embleton N, Collinson A, Menson E, Russell AB, Heath P. Missed opportunities for preventing group B streptococcus infection. Arch Dis Child - Fetal Neonatal Ed. 2010;95(1):F72-3.

46. Kuhn P, Dheu C, Bolender C, Chognot D, Keller L, Incidence and distribution of pathogens in early-onset neonatal sepsis in the era of antenatal antibiotics. Pediatr Perinat Epidemiol. 2010;24(5):479-87.

47. Verani JR, McGee L, Schrag SJ. Prevention of perinatal group B streptococcal disease. MMWR Recomm Rep. 2010;59(RR10):1-32.

48. Phares CR, Lynfield R, Farley MM, Mohle-Boetani J, Harrison LH, Petit S, et al. Epidemiology of Invasive Group B Streptococcal Disease in the United States, 1999-2005. JAMA. 2008;299(17):2056-65.

49. Verani JR, McGee L, Sharg SJ. Prevention of perinatal Group B streptococcal disease; revised guidelines from CDC, 2010. MMWR. 2010;59(RR10):1-32.

50. Brady MT, Polin RA. Prevention and Management of Infants With Suspected or Proven Neonatal Sepsis. Pediatrics. 2013;132(1):166-8.

51. Gras-Le Guen C, Foix-L'Helias L, Boileau P. Precocious neonatal bacterial infection (PNBI): which management algorithm in 2017?. Arch Ped. 2017;24:S14-7.

52. [No Authors listed]. Prevention of Early-onset Neonatal Group B Streptococcal Disease: Green-top Guideline No. 36. BJOG. 2017;124(12):e280-305.

53. Money D, Allen VM - Prevention of early-onset neonatal group B streptococcal infection. J Obstet Gynaecol Can. 2018;40(8):e675-86.

54. Six A, Joubrel C, Tazi A, Poyart C. Maternal-lacental infections with Streptococcus agalactiae. Presse Med. 2014;43(6):706-14.

55. Van Dyke MK, Phares CR, Lynfield R, Thomas AR, Arnold KE, Craig AS, et al. Evaluation of Universal Antenatal Screening for Group B Streptococcus. N Engl J Med. 2009;360(25):2626-36.

56. Ohlsson A, Shah VS. Intrapartum antibiotics for known maternal Group B streptococcal colonization. Cochrane Database Syst Rev. 2014;(6):CD007467.

57. Williams M. RCOG guidance: early-onset neonatal GBS disease. Prescriber. 2018;29(1):34-6.

58. Baker CJ, Byington CL, Polin RA. Policy statement-Recommendations for the prevention of perinatal group B streptococcal (GBS) disease. Pediatrics. 2011;128(3):611-6.

59. Polin RA, Newborn the COFA. Management of Neonates With Suspected or Proven Early-Onset Bacterial Sepsis. Pediatrics. 2012;129(5):1006-15.

60. Manning SD, Neighbors K, Tallman PA, Gillespie B, Marrs CF, Borchardt SM, et al. Prevalence of Group B Streptococcus Colonization and Potential for Transmission by Casual Contact in Healthy Young Men and Women. Clin

Infect Dis. 2004;39(3):380 - 8.

61. Foxman B, Gillespie BW, Manning SD, Marrs CF. Risk Factors for Group B Streptococcal Colonization: Potential for Different Transmission Systems by Capsular Type. Ann Epidemiol. 2007;17(11):854 - 62.

62. Boullevaux E. Efficience du mode de prélevement vaginal dans le cadre du depistage systématique du Streptocoque du groupe B: étude de 1353 prélevements. Available at: https://hal.univ-lorraine.fr/hal-01887614, accessed 01 June 2019.

63. OMS. Group B streptococcus vaccine development technology roadmap: priority activities for development, testing, licensure and global availability of group B streptococcus vaccines. Geneva: Word Health Organisation; 2017.

64. Ben Hamida Nouaili E, Abidi K, Chaouachi S, Marrakchi Z. Epidemiology of maternal-fetal group B streptococcal infections. Medecine Mal Infect. 2011;41(3):123-5.

65. Creti R, Imperi M, Berardi A, Pataracchia M, Recchia S, Alfarone G, et al. Neonatal Group B Streptococcus Infections. Pediatr Infect Dis J. 2017; 36(3): 256-62.

66. Rao GG, Nartey G, McAree T, O'Reilly A, Hiles S, Lee T, et al. Outcome of a screening programme for the prevention of neonatal invasive early-onset group B Streptococcus infection in a UK maternity unit: an observational study. BMJ Open. 2017;7(4):e014634.

<u>Telephone</u> :

<u>EVALUATION FORM FOR THE CARRIAGE OF STREPTOCOCCUS</u>
<u>OF THE</u>
<u>GROUP B AFTER 33 SA</u>

Number :   Date :   /   /

Name: Age :

Origin :

Level of education : Primary ◊ Secondary ◊ Higher ◊

Gestite :   Parite :   Profession   :

Weight :   Size   :

<u>ANTECEDENTS:</u>

Diabetes ◊ Neonatal death ◊
Spontaneous miscarriage ◊

Extrauterine pregnancy ◊

Acute pyelonephritis in pregnancy ◊

Death per partum ◊

Voluntary termination of pregnancy ◊

Threat of premature delivery^

Frequent in utero death ◊

Carriage of streptococcus B ◊

<u>PARAMETERS OF THE CURRENT PREGNANCY :</u>

Term of delivery: DDR :

Twin pregnancies ◊

Gestational diabetes ◊ Balance: Yes ◊ No ◊

Threat of premature delivery ◊ aSA

Acute pyelonephritis ◊

HTA g :

<u>WORK-RELATED PARAMETERS:</u>

On admission: Not in labour ◊ Latent phase ◊ Active phase ◊

Working hours :

Premature rupture of membranes ◊:   hours/partum

Antibiotics received: Type :

Total in g :

Febrile episode > a 38.5: ◊

Delivery: vaginal delivery ◊ vaginal delivery ◊ :- hot

-cold

<u>NEW PARAMETERS :</u>

APGAR at 5 min :

Birth weight :

Evolution: complications :

<u>MICROBIOLOGICAL PARAMETERS :</u>

Collection : Before admission ◊ On admission ◊

Direct examination :

☐ Sprout :

""--"--"--"--"--"--"--"--"--"--"--"--"--"--"--"--"--"--"--"-I

☐ Leukocytes :

☐ Associated pathogens :

Culture :

☐ Germ identified :

☐ Antibiogram :

Sensitive	Intermediate	Resistant

Decision-making scheme for GBS carriage screening and AIP (66)

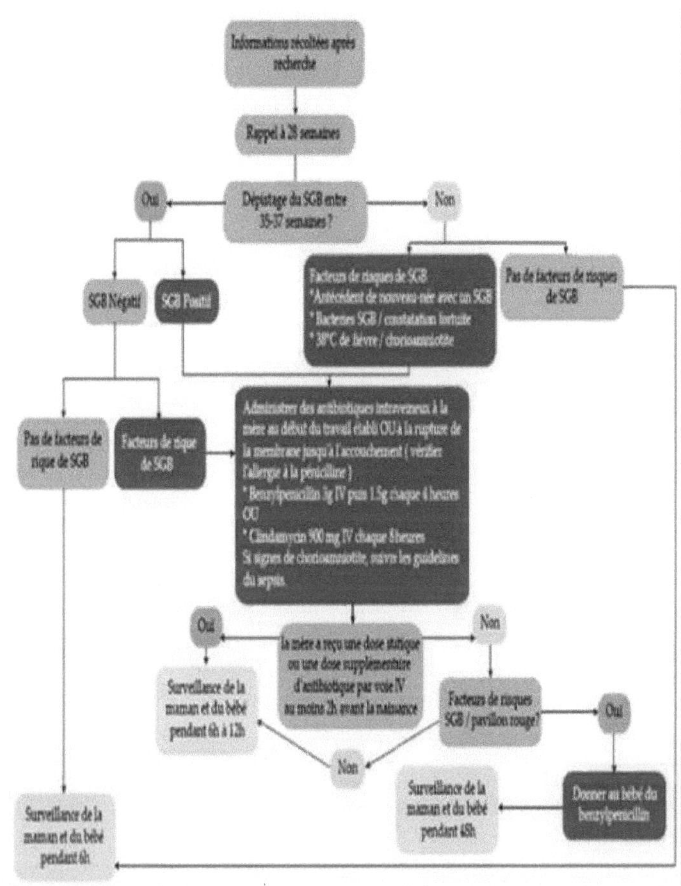

53

SCREENING FOR GENITAL CARRIAGE OF
GROUP B STREPTOCOCCUS
IN PREGNANT WOMEN IN THE
THIRD TRIMESTER

Resume

The last trimester of pregnancy is a period of high rates of genital carriage of germs at risk of maternal and neonatal infection. GBS is the most common germ. It is transmitted by the ascending route or through the vaginal passageway.

The objectives of our study were:

To determine the prevalence of vaginal carriage of streptococcus B in the third trimester of pregnancy.

Identify the main risk factors involved in portage.

Defining a screening strategy for streptococcus B.

To determine the diagnostic and therapeutic means of vaginal carriage of GBS. A cross-sectional study was carried out in the Obstetric Gynecology Department of the Fattouma Bourguiba University Hospital in Monastir, including 330 pregnant women in their third trimester who were screened from 34 weeks' gestation onwards, and women carrying streptococcus B were given appropriate antibiotic prophylaxis when they went into labour.

The portage rate was 8.8%.

This rate was significantly associated with antecedent diabetes and living in a rural environment.

Intapartum antibiotic prophylaxis was administered in 75.8% of patients who tested positive for GBS. 13.8% of newborns born to GBS-positive mothers were hospitalised; none were colonised.

Training healthcare teams and supporting them in implementing screening protocols and multidisciplinary neonatal management are essential to their success and effectiveness.

Keywords :	***Pregnancy-streptococcus B; Vaginal carriage; Screening; Risk factors; Prevalence; Antibiotic prophylaxis***

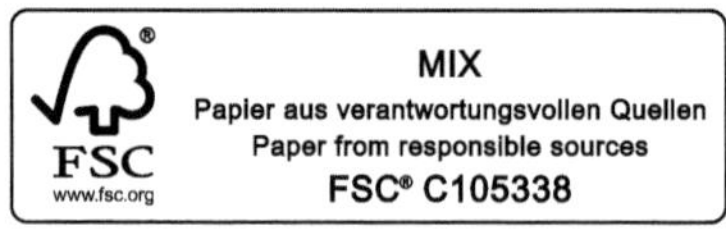

Printed by Books on Demand GmbH, Norderstedt / Germany